Keto No Bake Treats for Two Weeks:

A 14 Day Guide to Keto No-Bake Dessert Recipes

Introduction

I want to thank you and congratulate you for buying the book, "Keto No Bake Treats for Two Weeks: A 14-Day Guide to Keto No-Bake Dessert Recipes."

There is nothing that brings a smile to a face like a heavenly piece of dessert right after a meal. For most of us, it is the favorite part of a meal and the part that we all look forward to.

But, most of us feel the need to avoid taking desserts once we adopt a healthy low-carb diet like the keto diet. The good news is that not all desserts have to be too high in carbohydrates as you think. There are actually healthy keto-friendly desserts you can try out. If you are worried about baking and don't like how long it takes, then worry not because this book will focus on tasty, no-bake desserts.

Thanks again for getting this book, I hope you enjoy it!

The Basics

Before we learn some ketogenic desserts you can make, let us first understand what the ketogenic diet is. A ketogenic diet is basically a lifestyle of eating where you eat meals that are high in fat, very low in carbs and moderate in protein. This diet usually involves drastically reducing your carbohydrate intake and replacing the reduction with fats. That reduction then leads your body into a metabolic state of ketosis, which is the main goal for a ketogenic diet. You will learn why later on in the book.

As a beginner, the basic thing that you need to know about the ketogenic diet is that it makes your body very efficient at burning fat for fuel instead of carbohydrates. But how does it do that? Below is a breakdown of how the ketogenic diet works.

How The Ketogenic Diet Works?

When you eat a meal that is rich in carbohydrates, your body does two things.

- First, it takes those carbohydrates and converts them into glucose because glucose is the easiest molecule that your body can use as energy.

- Secondly, it produces insulin to move the glucose around your bloodstream and into your cells that need energy.

Since your body uses glucose as its primary source of energy, your alternative source of energy (fat) is. Therefore, what your body does is it stores the fat in your liver and muscle tissue as back-up energy source that your body can turn to when it is starved of its primary source of energy (glucose). The storing of fat normally leads to weight gain.

With the ketogenic diet, things are a bit different. As you now know, when you are on a ketogenic diet your intake of carbohydrate is at a minimum low. What that does to your body is it induces your body into a metabolic state of ketosis.

Ketosis is simply a natural process that your body initiates to help you survive when you are low on energy. In this process, your body tries to seek another form of energy source to utilize. It does that by making your liver convert fatty acids to ketone bodies, which give you an alternative energy source. With the ketogenic diet, your body normally runs on the fat that you consume and ketone bodies that it creates.

So why is ketogenic diet the best diet?

First, with the ketogenic diet, you reduce your carbohydrate intake, which makes your body to burn fat for energy; this usually leads to weight loss.

Secondly, optimum ketone levels in your body offers you many health benefits. Let's check out some of these benefits below;

It improves your mental health

When your body runs on ketone bodies, the health of your brain improves significantly because ketones are more energy efficient. Here is how? Your brain normally can't absorb glucose directly as energy. It usually has to wait for the glucose to be converted into a usable form of energy by your body.

Meanwhile, it has a protective feature that is known as blood brain barrier that stops unwanted materials including glucose from reaching it through the blood. So when you feast on foods rich in carbohydrates your brain usually gets drained trying to prevent the increase of glucose from getting into it before the glucose is converted into a usable form of energy. This mostly leads to you having afternoon crashes, mental fogs and slumps.

Ketone bodies are efficient because they can be used by your brain immediately after they have been produced. That automatically saves you mental fog and slumps that affect the health of your brain.

It fights and improves various health conditions and diseases

The other major benefit that you get from your body using ketones for energy is the improvement of various health conditions. Below are some of the illnesses that the ketogenic diet can help you improve and fight.

Type 2 diabetes: Type 2 diabetes is a health condition where your body becomes insulin resistant which means your cells don't respond to insulin. The condition makes it hard for your body to transport glucose to your cells and lower your high blood sugar levels, which are dangerous to your body as they can burst your veins open.

The Ketogenic diet helps you prevent and fight off type 2 diabetes by switching your body from depending on glucose for energy to depending on fats for energy. The diet limits your intake of glucose, which automatically lowers your blood sugar levels. That gets rid of the danger that insulin resistance poses to your body.

Polycystic Ovary Syndrome (PCOS): PCOS is a condition that is caused by insulin resistance. This condition gives women a wide range of hormonal issues one of the major ones being infertility. As you have seen above, a ketogenic diet deals with insulin resistance by making you eat foods that are low on carbohydrates. That helps you avoid the danger of having high sugar levels in your blood when your cells are resistance to insulin.

Glut1 Deficiency Syndrome: This is a genetic metabolic disorder that is caused by the deficiency of GLUT1, which is a protein that is responsible for transporting glucose through the blood brain barrier. The symptoms of this condition include frequent seizures, having difficulty with movement and having developmental delays.

The Ketogenic diet helps you fight this condition because unlike glucose, ketones don't need GLUT1 protein to cross from your blood stream to your brain. This means this diet provides you with an energy source that you can use efficiently even if you are suffering from GLUT1 Deficiency Syndrome.

It increases and stabilizes your energy levels

One of the downsides of following a diet rich in carbohydrates is the fact that you will have inconsistent energy levels. This is because your body can only store so much glucose as glycogen in your body. One way or the other you will need to refuel your energy and that creates a scenario of inconsistent energy levels.

This all changes when you follow a ketogenic diet. As you now know when you are in ketosis, your body runs on stored fat, which is in plenty in your body. This abundant supply of fat is what gives you stable energy levels in your body that never runs out.

As you can see, the ketogenic diet is a very beneficial diet that not only improves your health but also protects you from illnesses. That is what makes it ideal.

Let us now break it down further, and learn how to follow the ketogenic diet.

How to Follow the Ketogenic Diet?

Following the ketogenic diet is pretty simple, all you have to do is to make sure that your meals are high in fat, moderate in protein and low in carbohydrates. However, how low or high should your nutrient intake be?

The standard nutrient intake in a ketogenic diet is taking in a meal that is made up of **70% fat, 25% proteins and 5% carbohydrates.** If your goal is to lose weight, then the lower you make your carbohydrate intake the better the result you get.

To help you get started, here is a ketogenic eating routine that you can adopt.

Day 1

Breakfast: Fried eggs with mushrooms and bacon

Lunch: Guacamole salad with a handful nuts and celery sticks

Dinner: Salmon with asparagus

Day 2

Breakfast: Scrambled eggs with spinach

Lunch: Chicken salad with basil balsamic vinaigrette

Dinner: Fish and spinach cooked in coconut oil

Day 3

Breakfast: Strawberry smoothie

Lunch: Ham and cheese slices

Dinner: Pork chops with broccoli and Parmesan cheese

Having understood how the keto diet works, let us now learn if desserts are great for you

Is Dessert Good For You?

Before you get to know how you can prepare a delicious dessert, it is very important for you as a beginner to ask yourself one important question. Is dessert good for your health?

In most cases, dessert is normally seen as an unhealthy meal and for good reasons I might add. One of the good reasons why dessert is considered unhealthy is because majority of desserts are high in fat, sugar, processed carbohydrates and calories, which are factors that promote weight gain and the illnesses that comes with it such as diabetes and cardiovascular diseases like stroke and heart attacks. Therefore, even as you take the bold step of getting started on the ketogenic diet, you may feel stuck because you cannot eat such desserts; hence, the need to be creative.As a dessert lover that is not easy to hear but there is actually a silver lining.

So back to the question that is the topic of this chapter. Is dessert good for your health?

The answer is yes and no. Yes, dessert can be bad for your health and no it doesn't have to be because just like there are healthy and unhealthy foods, desserts can be unhealthy and can be made to be healthy. Let us learn some healthy deserts you can prepare at home.

Two Weeks No Bake Dessert Recipes

Below are some of the best dessert recipes below.

Chocolate Coconut Balls

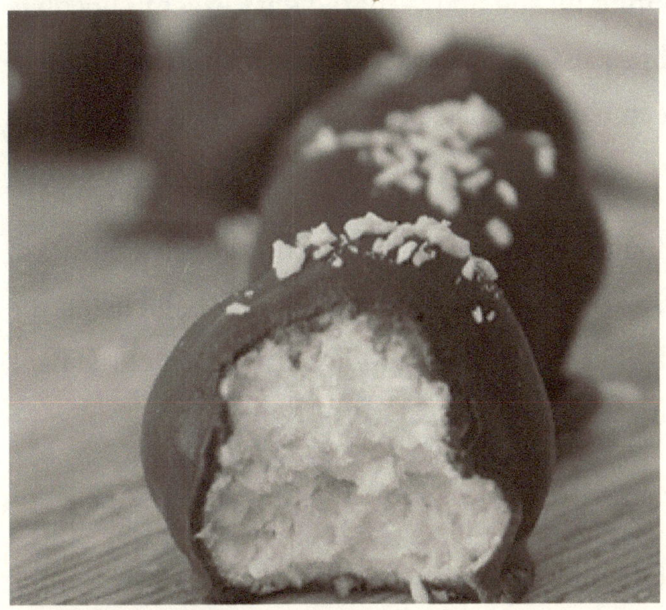

Makes 40 balls

Calories: 40

Proteins: 1g, Carbohydrates: 3g, Fats: 4g

Ingredients

1-2 cups of chocolate chips of your choice

¼ cup of coconut milk

¾ cup of sticky sweetener of choice

1 cup of blanched almond flour

3 cups of finely shredded coconut, unsweetened

Directions

Start by combining all the above ingredients except chocolate chips in a food processor or blender until it forms thick dough. If the dough becomes too thick, add an extra liquid of choice to lessen its thickness.

Transfer the dough into a large mixing bowl and lightly wet your hands. Use your wet hands to form small balls using the dough. Place the balls on a plate and into a fridge. Let the balls chill and firm up.

Meanwhile, prepare the chocolate by melting it. Set aside.

Remove the coconut balls from the fridge and start dipping each ball into the chocolate. Repeat the process until all the balls are evenly coated. Place the balls on a plate and into the fridge. Let the balls freeze further and become firmer.

Serve and enjoy.

Chocolate Cheesecake

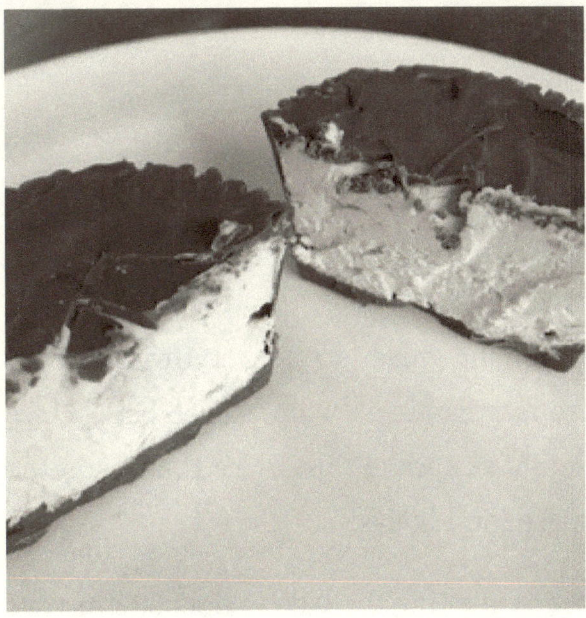

Serves 4

Calories: 323.75

Proteins: 4.25g, Carbohydrates: 5.25g, Fats: 29 g

Ingredients

Ganache

Splash of water

½ cup of heavy whipping cream

2 ounces of unsweetened baker chocolate

Cheesecake filling

¼ cup of erythritol

¼ cup of heavy whipping cream

2 tablespoon of sour cream

4 ounces of cream cheese

Directions

Make the filling: Use a hand mixer to mix erythritol, heavy whipping cream and sour cream in a medium sized bowl. Once done, dollop the filling into cupcake tins. Place the tins in the fridge and let them freeze for 2 hours.

Prepare ganache: Start by melting the baker chocolate in your microwave. Remove and add in heavy whipping cream. Mix the two ingredients until well combined. Add in splash of water and mix the mixture further until a thick liquid consistency is formed.

Make the chocolate cheesecake: Remove the cupcake tins from the fridge and pour ganache mix over them. Serve and enjoy.

Chocolate Fudge

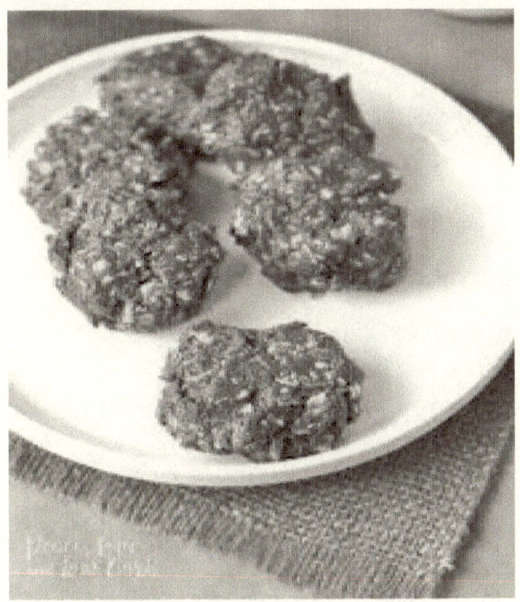

Serves 12

Calories: 172

Proteins: 2g, Carbohydrates: 1.5g, Fats: 18g

Ingredients

1 teaspoon of sugar free vanilla extract

1/3 cup of chopped walnuts

1 cup of unsweetened desiccated or shredded coconut

1/8th teaspoon of coarse sea salt or kosher salt

¼ cup of premium unsweetened cocoa powder

¾ cup of erythritol sweetener

½ cup of softened unsalted butter

4 ounces of softened cream cheese

Directions

Start by creaming butter, cocoa powder, sweetener and cheese until smooth. Use a fork or a mixer.

Add in vanilla extract, walnuts, coconut and salt. Stir the mixture well.

Spoon the mixture into 1 inch balls. You can enjoy the fudge right away or let the fudge chill for 30 minutes.

Keto Bars

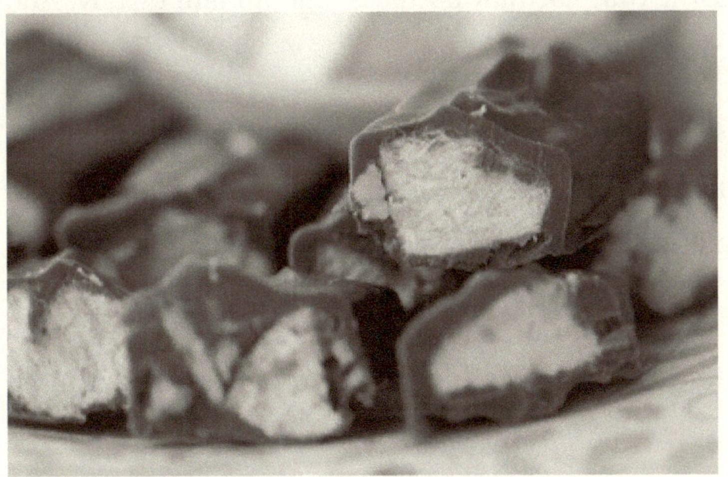

Makes 20 bars

Calories: 111

Proteins: 1g, Carbohydrates: 5g, Fats: 11g

Ingredients

2 cups of chocolate chips

2 ½ cups of unsweetened shredded coconut

¼ cup of sticky sweetener of choice

1 cup of melted coconut butter

Directions

Use a stovetop or a microwave-safe bowl to combine sticky sweetener with coconut butter. Place the mixture in a microwave and let it melt until smooth and creamy. Ignore the heating part if your coconut butter is smooth and drippy. Add in the coconut flakes and mix.

Line an 8 by 8 inch pan using parchment paper. Pour the coconut mixture into the lined pan and press it down until firmly in place. Transfer it to a refrigerator and let it chill until firm.

Remove from the fridge and cut the coconut mixture into 20 bars. Set aside.

Melt the chocolate chips and dip the 20 coconut bars into the chocolate mixture one chocolate bar at a time until well coated. Refrigerate the bars until they are firm. Serve.

Lemon Pudding

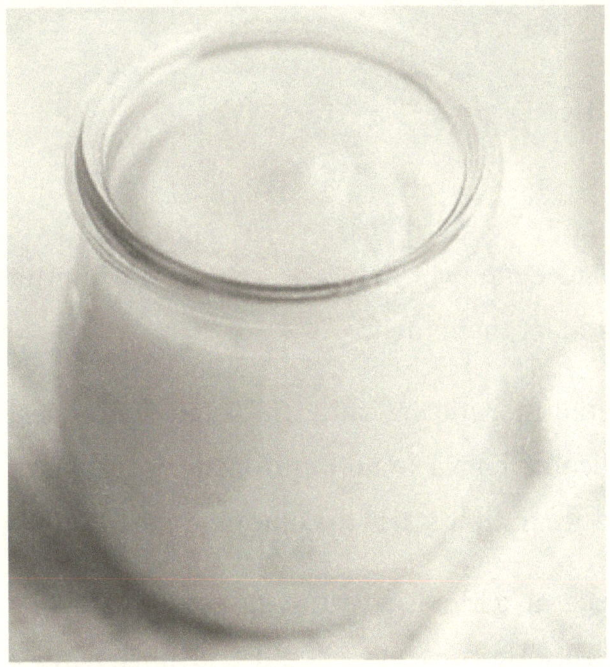

Serves 2

Calories: 412

Proteins: 7g, Carbohydrates: 3g, Fats: 41g

Ingredients

1/8 teaspoon of xanthan Gum

15 drops of liquid Stevia

½ juice lemon

1 teaspoon of lemon zest

4 large egg yolks

2 ounces of cream cheese

4 tablespoons of butter

Directions

Start by placing a saucepan over low heat. Add in your butter and cream cheese and let them melt.

While the ingredients melt down, shred in some lemon zest followed by the juice of half a lemon and lastly 15 drops of Stevia. Stir the mixture until it starts to come together.

Add in 1 yolk of egg at a time as you continue stirring the mixture with a whisk. The mixture should end up having a smooth and creamy texture.

Let the mixture cook further for a couple of minutes before you add in xanthan gum. Combine.

Pour the mixture into a bowl and cover the bowl loosely with a plastic wrap. Place the bowl in the fridge and let it chill for 2 hours.

Jello Mousse

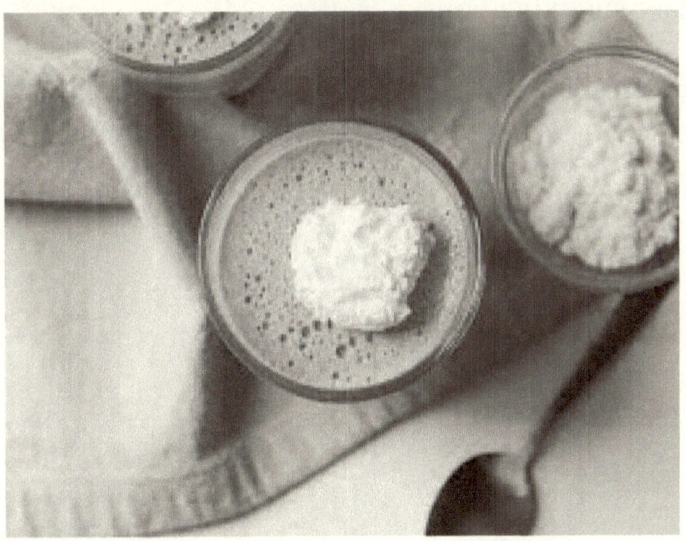

Serves 4

Calories: 97

Proteins: 20g, Carbohydrates: 3g, Fats: 3g

Ingredients

2 scoops of unflavored whey or just any other unflavored protein powder

10 ounces of plain Greek yogurt

½ cup of water

1 small box of sugar free black cherry Jello

Directions

Use a medium sized pan to heat up ½ cup of water until warm. The water shouldn't boil.

Place the sugar-free jello mix into a mixing bowl and pour the warm water over it. Let it sit as you organize the other ingredients.

Pour 2 scoops of protein powder and Greek yogurt into the mixing bowl with jello. Blend the mixture until smooth.

Transfer the mixture between 4 ramekins and let it sit for a few minutes.

Serve and enjoy.

Vanilla Smoothie

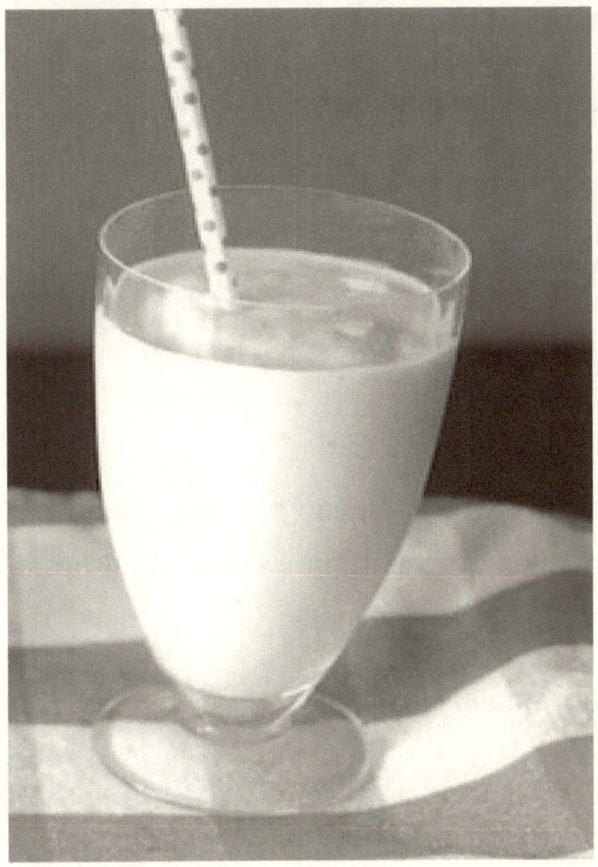

Serves 1

Calories: 566

Proteins: 34.6g, Carbohydrates: 5.1g, Fats: 45.2g

Ingredients

¼ cup of water

½ cup of ice

3-5 drops of Stevia extract

1 teaspoon of vanilla extract or 1 vanilla bean

1 tablespoon of extra virgin coconut oil or MCT oil

¼ cup of vanilla or plain whey protein

½ cup of coconut milk or soured cream

1-2 tablespoons of chia seeds or 2 large eggs

Directions

Place a mixture of vanilla extract, ¼ cup of water, plain whey protein, 2 eggs, sour cream, extra virgin coconut oil, drops of Stevia extract and ½ cup of ice in a blender.

Pulse the mixture until smooth.

Pour the mixture in a glass and serve immediately.

Blackberry Fat Bombs

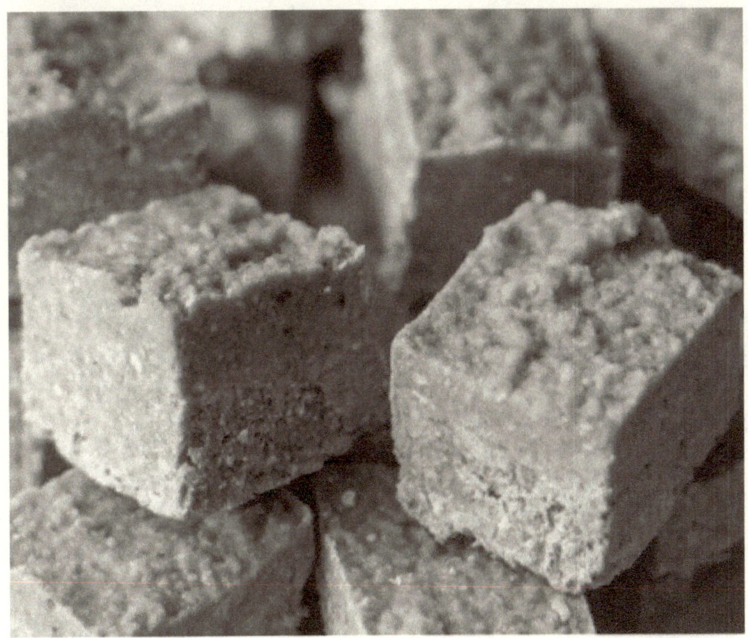

Makes 16 pieces

Calories: 170

Proteins: 1.1g, Carbohydrates: 3g, Fats: 18.7g

Ingredients

1 tablespoon lemon juice

½ teaspoon vanilla extract or ¼ teaspoon vanilla powder

½ teaspoon of Sweet Leaf stevia drops

½ cup of frozen or fresh blackberries.

1 cup of coconut oil

1 cup of coconut butter

Directions

Pour coconut oil, blackberries (if frozen) and coconut butter in a medium sized pot over medium heat. Let the ingredients heat up until well combined. Let the mixture cool for a minute or so.

Transfer the coconut oil mix in a food processor and add in the remaining ingredients; pulse until smooth.

Line a 6X6 inch container with parchment paper. Spread out the coconut and blackberry mixture onto the lined container. Refrigerate the mixture for an hour or until it hardens.

Remove the container from the fridge and place it upside down in a clean surface for the hardened mixture to separate itself from the container. Slice into squares.

Serve immediately or cover and store in the fridge.

AVOCADO POPSICLES

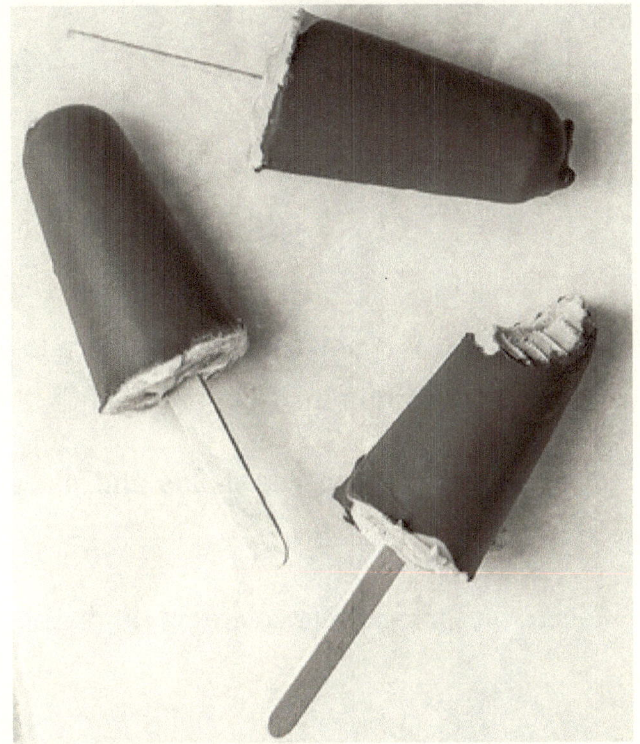

Serves 6

Calories: 33

Proteins: 1g, Carbohydrates: 2g, Fats: 1g

Ingredients

1 cup of unsweetened Almond milk

6 tablespoons of sugar alternative

2 tablespoons of lemon juice

2 medium avocados

Chocolate Ganache

2 teaspoons of Cacao butter

3 ounces of low carb chocolate

Directions

Start by mixing sugar alternative, lemon juice and 2 avocados in a mixer until everything is well combined.

Transfer the avocado mixture into Popsicle molds and place them in the freezer to freeze.

Meanwhile, melt Cacao butter and chocolate in a double container.

Remove the ice pops from the fridge and dip each one of them into the melted and slightly cooled chocolate. The chocolate shouldn't be too hot as it will melt the popsicle.

Enjoy immediately. Store the remaining pops in a freezer until ready to consume.

Cheesecake Mousse

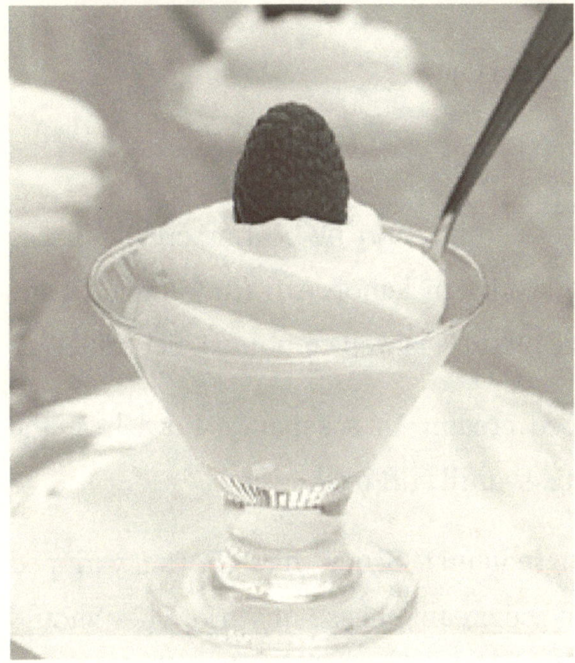

Serves 6

Calories: 269

Proteins: 3.7g, Carbohydrates: 16.5g, Fats: 27.8g

Ingredients

1 cup of heavy whipping cream

¼ teaspoon of lemon extract

1 ½ teaspoons of vanilla extract

1/8 teaspoon of stevia concentrated powder

1/3 cup of powdered erythritol or powdered low carb sweetener

8 ounces of softened cream cheese

Directions

Prepare the cream cheese mix: Start by beating cream cheese in a bowl until smooth. Mix in lemon extract, vanilla, Stevia and erythritol until the mixture is well combined. Set aside.

Prepare heavy whipped cream: In a separate bowl beat the heavy cream with a mixer until stiff peak forms.

Combine the two ingredients: Scoop half of the whipped cream and fold it into the cream cheese mixture. They should be well incorporated. Scoop the remaining half of the whipped cream and fold into the incorporated mixture.

Beat the mix using an electric mixer on high until light and fluffy. Refrigerate the mixer for two hours.

Spoon the mousse into serving dishes and top with sugar free chocolate or fresh fruit if desired.

Strawberry Cream Pie

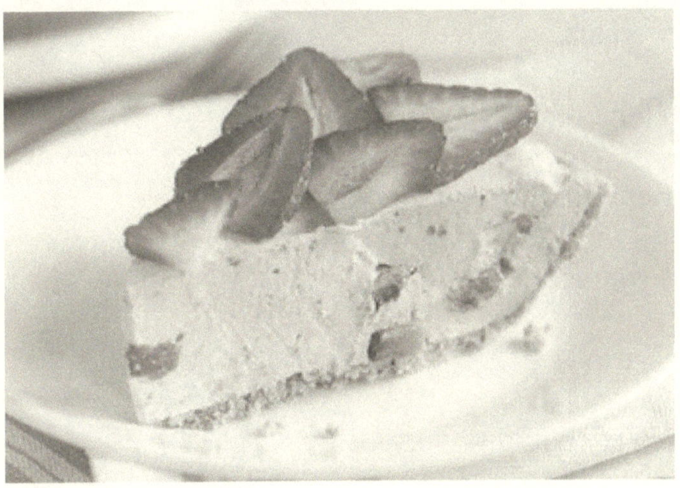

Serves 12

Calories: 368

Proteins: 5g, Carbohydrates: 7g, Fats: 36g

Ingredients

Crust

¼ cup of softened butter

¼ teaspoon of salt

1 cup of shredded unsweetened coconut

1 cup of unsalted raw sunflower seeds

Filling

2 tablespoons of water

½ cup of heavy cream

1 tablespoon of lemon juice

8 ounces of softened cream cheese

4 ounces of strawberries

1 teaspoon of gelatin

¼ teaspoon of Berry liquid stevia

3rd Layer

8 ounces of sliced strawberries

Toppings

2 cups of heavy cream

½ teaspoon of vanilla liquid stevia

Directions

Prepare the crust: Start by placing all the crust ingredients in your food processor. Switch the power on and pulse the mixture until it achieves the consistency of fine crumbs.

Oil a 10-inch spring-form pan and immediately spread crust ingredients at the bottom of the pan.

Prepare the filling: In a small saucepan, pour in water followed by a sprinkle of gelatin. Place the saucepan over low heat and let the mixture boil. Stir constantly as the mixture heats up. Keep on stirring until the gelatin dissolves completely.

Add in all the other filling ingredients except heavy cream in your food processor and pulse until smooth. Transfer the filling mixture into a stand mixer and add in heavy cream. Mix on high. The mixture should be whipped.

Add the cooled gelatin and blend it in for about a minute. Transfer and spread the mixture into the spring-form pan to form a second layer that is above the crust.

Place a third layer. Spread the sliced strawberries over the filling.

Prepare the topping. Add vanilla crème sweet drops and heavy cream into your stand mixer and pulse until whipped. Taste to adjust the sweet drops to your liking.

Smear the topping on top of the strawberries and spread until evenly distributed.

Refrigerate the pie for 2-3 hours or let the pie chill overnight.

Remove from the fridge. Make 12 slices and serve.

Ginger Cookies

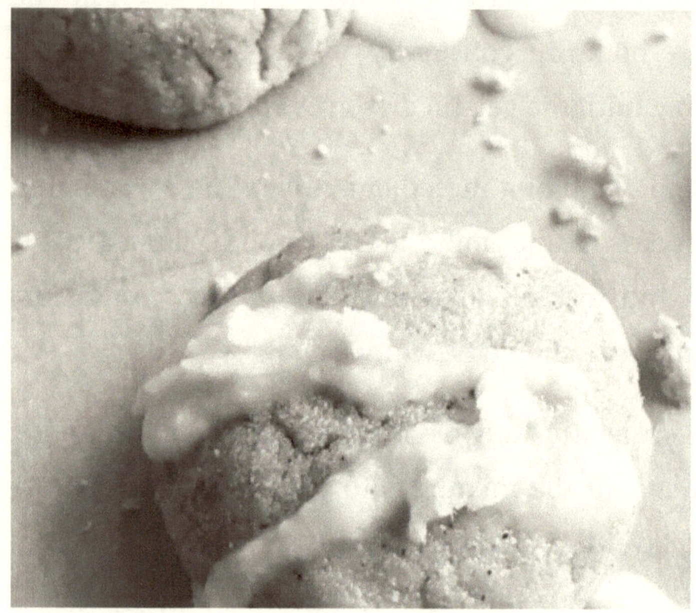

Serves 4

Calories: 157

Proteins: 6g, Carbohydrates: 7.5g, Fats: 12g

Ingredients

¼ teaspoons of freshly grated ginger (for garnish)

1 teaspoon of ground ginger

1 tablespoon of melted coconut butter

1 tablespoon of brain octane oil

2 vanilla shortbread collagen protein bars

Directions

Place ground ginger, Brain Octane and Collagen bars in a food processor. Pulse until the mixture forms a consistency that looks doughy than crumbly.

Slowly scoop a spoonful of the dough and place it in your palms. Form a round cookie by pressing the dough in between your palms. Repeat this process with the rest of the dough. You should end up with only round cookies.

Sprinkle the just formed cookies with coconut butter and garnish with freshly grated ginger.

Serve immediately or store in the fridge until you are ready to consume.

Vanilla Ice Cream

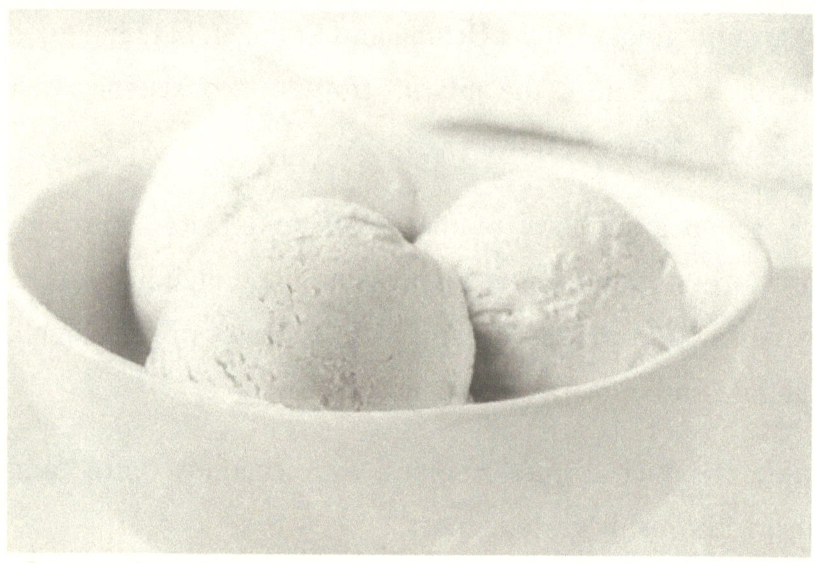

Serves 1

Calories: 408

Proteins: 2g, Carbohydrates: 3g, Fats: 46g

Ingredients

1/3 cup of salt

4 cups of ice

1 tablespoon of erythritol or any sweetener of your choice

1/8 teaspoon of minced vanilla bean

½ teaspoon of vanilla extract

½ cup of heavy cream

Directions

Start by placing a mixture of erythritol sweetener, vanilla bean, vanilla extract and heavy cream in a medium sized bowl. Mix everything together using a hand mixer. Pour the mixture into a zippered sandwich bag and zip it up to close.

Take a gallon size freezer bag and add in 1/3 cup of salt and 4 cups of ice. Now place the zippered sandwich bag into the gallon size freezer bag and close.

Give the gallon size freezer bag a good shake for 6-10 minutes or until you get your preferred ice cream firmness. Shake some more if you want a firmer ice cream. Once done, open the gallon size bag and remove the sandwich freezer bag.

Use cool water to carefully rinse the closed sandwich bag. This helps you get the salty water off the bag. Lack of rinsing the salt can give your ice cream a salty taste. Place the bag on the freezer and let it cool for 20 minutes- 1 hour depending on how firm you desire your ice cream to be.

Remove from the fridge, scoop into a bowl or a glass and enjoy.

Strawberry Chia Pudding

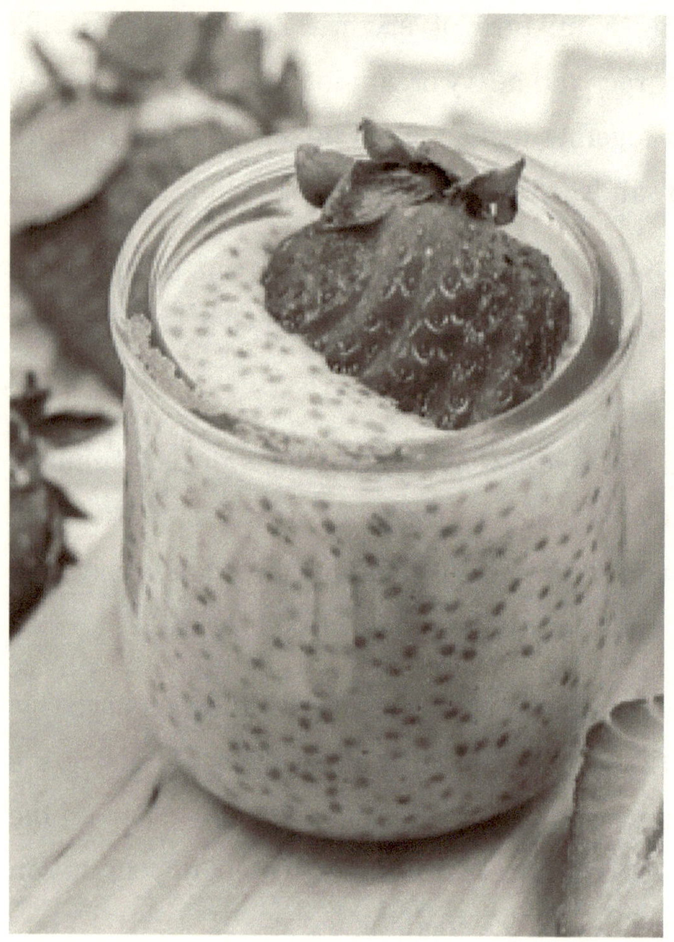

Serves 4

Calories: 111

Proteins: 4.4g, Carbohydrates: 10.8g, Fats: 1.8g

Ingredients

1 cup of frozen or fresh chopped strawberries

1 tablespoon of lemon juice

1/8 teaspoon of monk fruit liquid extract

1/8 teaspoon of vanilla stevia drops

1/3 cup of chia seeds

2 cups of unsweetened almond milk

Directions

Start by stirring chia seeds into almond milk in a medium sized bowl.

Add in strawberries, lemon juice and sweeteners. Mix all ingredients with a hand mixer until well combined. Stir the mixture every 5 minutes for 15 minutes.

Divide the mixture into serving dishes and place them on the fridge to chill for 4 hours or overnight.

Remove and enjoy the pudding.

Ketogenic Diet And Exercise

While the ketogenic diet is quite effective when it comes to weight loss, you will benefit a great deal by incorporating exercise. This is because when you work out, you burn more calories, which leads to weight loss. In addition, working out offers other benefits such as:

- A release of feel good hormones after a workout

- Strengthens your core

- Enables you to participate in physical activities without getting tired too fast

- Prevents certain diseases

The above are just examples of the benefits you stand to enjoy by working out. Therefore, don't neglect your physical activity.

If going to the gym is too much for you, you can opt for other forms of exercise such as swimming, dancing, doing yoga etc. just find that one thing that you enjoy and works for you and you are likely to stick with it in the long run.

Conclusion

Thank you again for buying this book!

I hope this book was able to help you to know that you can prepare tasty desserts even when on the ketogenic diet. The next step is to try these desserts and you will be amazed at how good they taste.

Finally, if you enjoyed this book, would you be kind enough to leave a review for this book on Amazon?

Thank you and good luck!

www.ingramcontent.com/pod-product-compliance
Lightning Source LLC
Chambersburg PA
CBHW051132250726
48655CB00007B/3010